BECOMING A CEO
OF SELF-CONFIDENCE

YOUR LITTLE *Blaque*
BOOK OF INNER STRENGTH

BY C. ZAKI ROSHELL

To stay up to date with
new products and get access to
free resources, visit zakiblaque.store

TABLE OF CONTENTS

FOREWORD

I have had the fortune to know Zaki her whole life. I met her when she was a baby, long before she became a fashion designer and CEO, and I've had the pleasure of watching her mature from a precocious young person to an intellectual thought leader. Every time I hear about one of her many accomplishments, I am more and more in awe of this young woman.

Reading Zaki's ideas on self-confidence and how it can shape your life is particularly intriguing to me. As someone who has started many businesses - some successful, some not so much - I value learning new concepts that can enhance my work and life. I wish I had a roadmap like this when I was getting started, and even at this stage in my career, I plan to take some of her advice!

Even though Zaki is much younger than I am and probably younger than many of you readers, I believe she is uniquely qualified to write this book. She has had a singular vision and passion, and she has more follow-through than many of the middle-aged professionals I deal with on a regular basis. There is power in the voice of the youth, and I invite you all to harness that power.

Vernard Hodges, DVM
CEO, Critter Fixer Veterinary Hospital
Star, "Critter Fixers: Country Vets"

DEDICATION

*This book is dedicated
to the continuous pursuit of self-love.*

INTRODUCTION

*H*ave you ever had a great idea but didn't tell anyone about *it*? Have you ever wanted to do something really big but didn't? Do you ever dream of stepping into your passion or taking an exciting risk but choose to play it safe instead?

A survey of 1,000 teens conducted by Wakefield Research shared that "many teens are interested in doing big things like chasing a dream, changing the world, or starting a business, but choose not to because the risks that come with these ideas are a major concern." "Fear of Failure" is a prime concern of 67 percent of teens, who say fear might stop them from following their passions.

I completely understand these statistics. It takes vulnerability and confidence to share a big idea, for which you might be judged. Exposing your passion to friends and family is one thing but declaring your ambitions to the world opens you up to an entirely different level of fear and anxiety.

Suppose you want to pursue a sports dream, attack a passion project, or start a business. In that case, many organizations and individuals can help you make these opportunities a reality. The problem, however, is that while they can support you in making your dreams a reality, if you lack self-confidence, you will always be afraid to move forward or take the next step. And there are very few organizations or resources geared toward helping young people like you and me develop the much-needed mindset of a visionary.

Your mindset is where it all begins. Self-confidence is the key to living life fearlessly and to the fullest.

My name is Zaki Roshell, and I am a teenage fashion designer from Douglasville, Georgia. I am the CEO of Zaki's Tutu Tops clothing boutique and Zaki Blaque, a brand specializing in tulle designs.

Other girls my age are wearing Gucci and Louis, and that's nice, but when I get asked "who you got on", I can say that I wear me!

My brand is all about strength, beauty, and confidence. When I walk into a room, it's clear that I am a CEO of total self-confidence. I believe in myself completely!

The book you are holding is the collection of strategies and information that became the guidebook I used to become the CEO of my self-confidence. Within these pages, you will discover the steps you can take to become responsible for your self-confidence and belief in yourself.

Before diving into the work, there are 3 things you must do to make everything else in the book possible. These three things will allow you to put your fears aside, get out of your own way, and level up.

First, you must acknowledge your fears.

What is it that you're afraid of? Why are you afraid? It's almost like confronting yourself when you ask yourself these things.

Try this exercise

Sit down, grab a pencil and paper and write down what you are afraid of. Identify it and create a plan

One tool I use every day is a planner. I use this to write down actions I want to take to move closer to what I want to achieve.

Secondly, it's important to practice building your self-confidence every day.

I like to think of self-confidence as a muscle; you must exercise it to build it and make it strong. The tips, tools, and strategies you will get in this book are just the beginning. There is no magic spell in these pages. You must take responsibility and do the work every day.

The final step I want you to take as you get ready to begin is to Embrace Your Journey.

Obtaining self-confidence will allow you to live life fearlessly, which may not always be easy. Be nice to yourself on your journey, but don't baby yourself.

There were times when I had to get on myself, like, "Okay, Zaki, you really need to do better, girl because this is not it."

Understand that there will always be other opportunities to show your progress because your self-confidence journey is a process. Show yourself grace. Always reflect, redirect, and keep moving forward. Don't ever compare your journey to someone else's journey. Stay in your lane and forge your own path.

When I launched my business, I would always compare myself to more established brands, and it caused me to lose sight of what I wanted my business to be. When I stepped back and realized that this was my journey, things began to fall into place.

Alright! So let's recap. Now that you're ready to start working on your confidence, remember to

1. Acknowledge your fears.

2. Practice and flex your self-confidence muscle every day.

3. Embrace your journey.

You are ready to begin if you've got those things locked and loaded. Let's go!

HOW TO USE THIS BOOK:

Take your time. There is no rush. Each lesson builds on the last, so work your way through each chapter. Take notes and highlight areas where you need to focus more than others. At the end of each chapter, there is an area to do a brain dump. This is a space to keep your notes, record your thoughts, and capture any ideas that arise as you read.

Some chapters will encourage you to reflect; others will motivate you to execute. Your main responsibility is to do the work and be your self-confidence CEO.

If you get stuck, reach out to someone you trust; a parent, teacher, church leader, counselor, or mentor. They will be able to give you feedback that might just help you get unstuck.

The last section will provide examples of the resources I present in the book. Use them as a way to get started right away while you look for a resource that fits your needs best.

I have also created a companion planner for this book. It's amazing and helps put everything you learn in this book into practice. You may purchase it at www.zakiblaque.com

Well, it's time. You are officially ready to become the CEO of your self-confidence. I will see you inside!

Love,

Zaki

Part 1

EVERYTHING YOU SHOULD KNOW ABOUT SELF-CONFIDENCE

"It is confidence in our bodies, minds, and spirits that allows us to keep looking for new adventures."
– Oprah Winfrey

Chapter 1

CONFIDENCE VS. SELF-CONFIDENCE

I am the CEO of Zaki Blaque and Zaki's Tutu Tops. A CEO is the Chief Executive Officer of a company or organization. This simply means that I am the head of my company. I am the person who makes the decisions that allow my team to plan and execute the dreams I have for my business.

Zaki Blaque is a fashion brand that specializes in custom looks, designs, and accessories. I started my brand when I was 16. I began by designing and creating luxurious Tutu tops. In the beginning, I was unsure of the way others would receive them, but when I began wearing my designs to various functions, the response I received from everyone was always exciting, and I always left with numerous requests for purchasing information. Over time, I decided that I was on to something special and I officially dived into manufacturing.

I remember the first time I was asked to view my first line of designs. I was excited and eager to see my dreams on display. While being a fashion designer and owner of my own clothing brand was something I had always hoped for, it was something I had never done. I was nervous and a little unsure. Yet even with the nerves, I believed that I could accept the challenge and deliver.

I relied on self-confidence to move forward and seize the moment. I will use the word self-confidence a lot in this book, so you need to know what it is and how it differs from confidence. Throughout my years as a student, teachers and leaders have really stressed the importance of having confidence or being confident. While I do believe confidence is important, I believe self-confidence is MORE important.

I define self-confidence as being secure in yourself and your abilities. Self-confidence is the emotional expression of trust and faith in yourself. Self-confidence often shows up in unwavering faith in your ability to take action, push past fear or uncertainty and accomplish what you want or need to accomplish. Self-confidence requires courage. Courage is the willingness to take action despite fear, uncertainty, or discomfort.

Confidence, on the other hand, is relying on previous experiences and finding security based on what you've been able to do or accomplish in the past. Confidence is using past experiences as evidence that you can do something rather than trusting that you are capable of doing something even if you've never done it before. Both confidence and self-confidence are important. However, if you only rely on what you've accomplished in the past, you will struggle to tackle new opportunities or new possibilities in the future.

Self-confidence doesn't just happen. It requires work and careful attention to develop strong and healthy self-confidence. You are the only person who can truly control your level of self-confidence. Teachers, friends, and leaders can provide tips, strategies, and resources like this book to help deepen or strengthen your self-confidence, but the work is up to you. By doing the work, you become a self-confident young woman who doesn't shy away from new possibilities and experiences because you confidently say "yes" when it's time to seize the moment.

As the CEO of your life, the main person responsible for planning and executing the life you desire, it is your responsibility to design a strong and healthy self-confidence intentionally. This book will guide you in accomplishing that goal, but it is up to you to make the important decisions and do the work.

Brain Dump

Chapter 1

How would you rate your self-confidence? (1-10)

_____

_____

_____

_____

_____

Notes, Thoughts, and Ideas

_____

_____

_____

_____

_____

Chapter 2

THE MYTHS ABOUT
SELF-CONFIDENCE

So, as you can see, self-confidence is pretty complex. At first glance, it can seem a little complicated or maybe even a little confusing, but understanding self-confidence is one of the greatest keys to accomplishing many of your greatest desires. In chapter 1, we defined self-confidence and how it differs from confidence. In this chapter, I want to clarify things by looking at what self-confidence is NOT.

If you were to ask someone to describe me, depending on whom you asked, they might describe me as reserved, organized, charismatic, fun, kind, or focused. I am true to all those things, but none of them is what makes me self-confident. None of those things define what self-confidence is or what it looks like. Self-confidence isn't about being awesome, having swag, or drippin' with finesse. It is about being your perfectly imperfect self.

Let's uncover a few other myths about what self-confidence is.

MYTH #1:
SELF-CONFIDENCE IS HAVING HIGH SELF-ESTEEM.

Self-confidence is not the same as self-esteem. Self-esteem is the belief that you are good enough. It is a general belief that you are worthy and valuable. While it is true that a person with high self-esteem will typically have healthy self-confidence, self-confidence (belief in what you can do) does not automatically mean having self-esteem (the belief that you are valuable). Self-esteem is really important and helpful when building your self-confidence, but they are not the same thing.

MYTH #2:
SELF-CONFIDENCE EQUALS BOLDNESS.

Being bold is a style. It is the way one approaches a situation or takes on a task. To be bold is to be daring, to be a risk-taker, or to be brave in the face of fear. Boldness is an excellent characteristic; it is a strong character trait, but boldness is not self-confidence. Like putting on a coat or a piece of jewelry, boldness is something you put on. Self-confidence is a belief; it is a part of who you are, not how you do something.

MYTH #3:
SELF-CONFIDENCE IS BEING FEARLESS.

Fearless literally means doing something without fear. Fearlessness sees fear as an obstacle to be conquered or overcome in the urgency to accomplish a task that might be risky or new. Like boldness, fearlessness is a characteristic, not a belief. Many individuals take on risky tasks because they want to accomplish a task. However, they do not have a belief in themselves that tells them that they will be successful. Many people with self-confidence have a healthy sense of fearlessness, but it is important to know that being afraid or cautious does not mean you lack self-confidence.

MYTH #4:
SELF-CONFIDENCE IS ARROGANCE.

Arrogance is an exaggerated sense of one's abilities. It is the belief that you are better, smarter, or more important than someone else because of your success or insecurities. Arrogance is always comparing oneself against another and determining their importance in relation to someone else. Self-confidence is not determined based on what anyone else does. Self-confidence comes from self-reflection and competing with yourself alone.

MYTH #5:
SELF-CONFIDENCE IS LOUD.

We often describe someone with a big personality, strong opinions, big facial expressions, and conversations that produce a great deal of sound as loud. Loudness describes a sound that is made not only with volume but also with the body. While knowing how to speak up and be heard is very important, being self-confident does not require high volume, and being loud does not mean that you believe in your ability to accomplish great things.

While it is true that many people believe that if you are loud, arrogant, fearless, or bold, you are self-confident, these characteristics and styles do not define or indicate that someone is self-confident. Self-confidence is personal. It is a belief; it is something only you know about yourself. Self-confidence does indeed produce behaviors that can be seen outwardly. A self-confident person will take risks. They are brave and daring, but these behaviors come from within, and a person with self-confidence isn't putting on a fake style to pretend to be something they are not.

Developing healthy self-confidence is important, and I will talk about why in the next chapter.

Brain Dump

Chapter 2

What myths have you believed about self-confidence?

_____

_____

_____

_____

_____

Notes, Thoughts, and Ideas

_____

_____

_____

_____

Chapter 3

DEVELOPING A HEALTHY
SELF-CONFIDENCE

I was 16 when I presented my first fashion show. I had seen fashion shows before and knew they required a lot of time and energy. At first, I was excited, but that excitement quickly turned to uncertainty as I considered everything that would have to go into hosting a fashion show. Not only would it require a large investment of money, but it would also require a great investment of time and energy.

Designers who host a typical fashion show spend, on average, 3-5 months planning and sketching hundreds of designs. Those designs are narrowed down to 30-40 looks, and then they spend 6-7 months working and bringing their designs to life. You must also consider the number of models needed and ensure each is perfectly measured so your designs look their best.

I considered all of these details and weighed the decision of whether or not I could do the show I was being asked to do. I took time to reflect and write down all the things that could go wrong. I journaled my fears and listed all the things that excited me about the opportunity. Once I had thought about all of those things, I began reviewing my knowledge and skills against my concerns. I thought about the routines and systems I had mastered and journaled exactly how they would help ensure some of my biggest fears or concerns didn't happen.

After taking the time to really evaluate the opportunity and reflect on my ability to accomplish the task successfully, I was able to say yes and get to work. I was sure of myself and had certainty in my ability to deliver. That is the power of self-confidence.

But self-confidence doesn't just happen. You can't just wake up one morning and be full of self-confidence. Healthy self-confidence is developed with purpose and intent. In this chapter, you will discover how you can begin the work of developing self-confidence.

The Question: How is self-confidence developed?

The Answer: Through Reflection and Routines.

Reflection is something we don't do enough of. Reflection is pausing to think about a situation and asking a series of questions while thinking. Effective reflection is done in a way that captures the answers to the questions you ask in a way that allows you to revisit them as often as necessary. That might be through keeping a journal or a diary.

Routines are a sequence of actions done the same way each time. When developing self-confidence, it is important to have routines you can lean on that help you organize yourself in a way that provides you with a strong foundation to start on.

As the CEO of your self-confidence, you must begin by developing some basic routines. These routines will become the foundation from which you start every task. These routines will allow you to become and feel more confident in yourself and your abilities.

Begin by capturing your thoughts. You may use the brain dump area at the end of this chapter. Next, find a quiet space where you feel safe being alone with your thoughts. Set a timer for 20 minutes and respond to these questions as honestly as possible. Don't worry about being judged, and don't judge yourself; just be honest.

Question #1: How do you feel when you are asked to do something new?

Question #2: What makes you nervous or insecure?

Questions #3: Are you organized? What areas of your life are the most organized? How do you keep those areas organized?

Question #4: What tasks do you do the same way every time you do them?

Question #5: What systems do you have to ensure things get done or don't fall through the cracks?

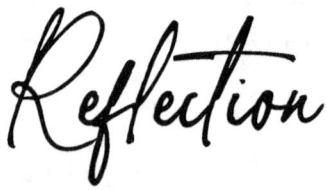

How do you feel when you are asked to do something new?

_____

_____

_____

What makes you nervous or insecure?

_____

_____

_____

What helps to keep you organized?

_____

_____

_____

What tasks do you do the same way every time you do them?

_____

_____

_____

What systems have you created for yourself?

_____

_____

_____

Brain Dump

Chapter 3

How often do you spend time reflecting?

_____

_____

_____

_____

_____

**Notes, Thoughts,
and Ideas**

_____

_____

_____

_____

_____

Chapter 4

BARRIERS TO
SELF-CONFIDENCE

I have a strong and healthy self-confidence, which I am very proud of, but I have not always felt this way. During my first year of Middle School, I began to feel a strong urge to do something great. I wanted to have an impact on my friends, family, and community. I shared my thoughts and dreams with my parents, who were excited about my passion. They encouraged me to explore this urge closely. They wanted me to clarify what this impact might look like and all of the various ideas I had.

As we explored these feelings together, we recognized that I would have to have a solid foundation to accomplish all my dreams. I would have to develop strategies for dealing with disappointment, overwhelm, and anxiety, so my mom enrolled me in a program for young ladies. The focus of the program was etiquette and self-esteem. During my time in this program, I learned a lot about myself as well as how to be the best version of myself, even in difficult situations.

As I gained more self-esteem and self-confidence, I began to keep a journal. This journal was almost like taking notes on my journey and the lessons I was learning. I noticed that I had many areas that required my full attention and other areas that came easily. Those areas that required my full attention were like barriers I had to overcome to develop strong self-confidence.

As we've discussed in previous chapters, self-confidence is the expectation that you can bring about a positive outcome to the things you want. It is the belief that you can accomplish your goals and know you have the skills necessary. Without healthy self-confidence, it becomes easy to procrastinate, resist change, and live in a constant state of sadness or anxiety. When you have self-confidence, you are happier and more willing to try new things.

While some of us have a strong and healthy self-confidence, many struggle in this area. We want to believe in ourselves, but sometimes we struggle to gain the self-confidence we desire. Many times, these barriers get in the way of developing self-confidence. As the CEO of your self-confidence, it is important to identify any barriers that may be getting in your way and do the work of removing them.

In this chapter, I will present some of the most common barriers to developing strong and healthy self-confidence. As you read them, ask yourself if you have experienced these barriers. If you do, circle the barrier, and begin thinking of ways to remove it. Use the journal pages in the back of this book to help you keep track of the barriers you identify and be intentional about working to remove them. If you need help, talk to someone you trust who can help you work through removing the barriers.

BARRIER #1: FAKING IT

Have you ever heard the saying, "Fake it until you make it?" While this idea isn't completely bad, the idea of "faking it" has become a big barrier to developing real and healthy self-confidence. Faking it until you make it can be a good strategy, especially if you're thrown into something at the last minute or want to seize a time-sensitive opportunity. However, it should only be used as a temporary strategy. The idea of faking it should not be your consistent way of living. When you are always pretending, you never fully develop a clear understanding of what you are good at.

Pretending is exhausting and can make you believe, subconsciously, that you really don't know what you're doing. Faking it stirs up anxiety and produces insecurity. When you pretend to know what or how to do things consistently, you create a barrier that prevents you from truly being self-confident.

How to remove this barrier: Show up as the real you!

Take time to identify your strengths. Describe them in detail and then record how those strengths impact other areas and tasks. For example, you may be a great writer. Depending on the parts of writing you excel in, you may have beautiful handwriting, you may have good research skills, you may be a good speller, or you may be great at organization and structure. These skills are useful in public speaking, art, editing, and studying. With this knowledge, you can confidently accept tasks that utilize these skills, and as you complete them using your real skills, you will no longer try to fake them. You will show up as the real you, and your self-confidence will grow.

BARRIER #2: FEAR

Many of us think of fear as bad, so we pretend not to be afraid or mask our fear, but fear is not bad. Fear is a useful emotion that works to get our attention. When we feel afraid, we tend to freeze. Instead, when we are afraid, we should pause to determine why our emotions are trying to get our attention. More often than not, our emotions are working to protect us from hurt, embarrassment, or disappointment. The feelings cause our brains to think of all the possible things that could go wrong. I once read that fear can be thought of as an acronym, FEAR: False Evidence Appearing Real.

While fear is a real emotion and can alert us to real danger, most of the time, the things that we are fearful of are the things we've created in our minds. You may be afraid of failing, or you may be afraid of being rejected or laughed at. You might even be afraid of what it will look like if you are successful. These imaginary pitfalls are not real; thinking of them as real can cause you to not believe in yourself and remain stuck.

How to remove this barrier: Speak to your fear!

When fear prevents your ability to believe in yourself, it's important to talk to your fear. Start by asking these questions:

Is this fear real? If it isn't real, or you know the fear is imaginary, repeat some strong affirmations and move forward. If the fear is real, ask yourself the next question.

How do you know this fear is real? Has this happened to me before?

If you're afraid of something that hasn't happened yet, pay attention to the fear, lean into it and ask yourself. What about this particular situation is making me the most afraid? Am I able to accomplish this task even though I'm afraid? What can I do to help address this fear in a way that can allow me to foresee any obstacles or setbacks? How might I be able to overcome any of the obstacles that I might experience?

If something has happened before and you are afraid it might happen again, evaluate the situation. Why did it happen? What did you learn? What can you do to prevent it from happening again?

Once you have asked and answered these questions, list out all of the skills, resources, and strategies you can use to ensure that you will be safe moving forward. Then move forward. If you are still fearful, do it scared!

BARRIER #3: PROCRASTINATION

Procrastination is the delay or postponement of something; it means putting off something that could be done now until later. Procrastination will rob you of self-confidence because it will keep you from being your best.

When you procrastinate and delay doing something until the last minute, you will find yourself under a constant weight of anxiety. Procrastination will always make you feel uneasy and keep you in a constant state of panic because you will always be in a rush. Every time you leave something to be done at the last minute, it will never be as good as it could have been.

Procrastination is a big obstacle to believing in yourself, making it hard for your self-confidence to grow.

How to remove this barrier: Make a plan!

If you're going to be the best version of yourself, the self-confident version, you want to be. You must learn to set boundaries, determine your priorities, and plan for success. When you take the time to do this, you can plan your tasks according to your priorities and the deadlines you have set, and you can create the boundaries that will allow you to do things according to the plan you create. Attending to your priorities and boundaries will help you plan better and give your best every time. When you give what you know is your best, your self-confidence blossoms, and that belief in yourself will become permanent.

BARRIER #4: STAYING IN YOUR COMFORT ZONE

Your comfort zone is the place or situation where you feel safe or at ease. It's the space where you experience the least amount of stress. We all love our comfort zone because we like to be in control. Our comfort zone is predictable, and everyone loves predictability.

When you are in your comfort zone, you're not stretching; if you're not stretching, you're not growing. In your comfort zone, you're maintaining the status quo. You're doing the little things that can be done with little effort.

This becomes a barrier to our self-confidence because we never put our abilities to work. We are never able to see what we are capable of, and when we are unsure of our capacity to do something challenging, we struggle to believe that we can.

How to remove this barrier: Do something new!

Take on a new challenge every month. Put your skills to the test and challenge yourself to learn new ones. When you know your abilities and strengths, you can stretch yourself to step outside of your comfort zone and see your skills used in different ways. As you see all the things you can do, your belief in yourself will grow, and your self-confidence will deepen.

BARRIER #5: DOING NOTHING

Self-confidence grows, and your belief in yourself gets stronger when you can see yourself accomplishing things you didn't know you could accomplish or accomplishing goals you set for yourself. The biggest barrier to developing strong self-confidence is doing nothing.

Just as it takes effort to become a better writer, get a good grade in math, make the cheerleading squad, make the track team, or get into the Beta Club, it also takes effort on your part to grow your self-confidence.

Oftentimes, however, because of the barriers I've mentioned above, we become frozen or stuck, and instead of taking an active role in our growth, we do nothing. Nothing happens when we do nothing, and when nothing happens, our self-confidence suffers.

How to remove this barrier: Reflect and Journal

Reflect on the times you felt most confident. Keep track of the moments when you feel the greatest belief in yourself.

What are those things that you do? Find ways to do more of those things, make time for them, and celebrate each time you succeed. When you take ownership of your own self-confidence, you will begin to grow in ways you never thought possible.

BARRIER #6: BLAME

Self-confidence is all about taking responsibility for your own behavior. This goes for the things we get right and the mistakes we make. When you credit someone else for the work you do by shrinking or playing small, you tell yourself that you are not capable of greatness, and your subconscious mind begins to believe that lie. When you blame others for your mistakes, by putting others at fault, you're never able to grow, you're never able to develop, and you're unable to identify the areas where you can grow.

How to remove the barrier: Take responsibility for your actions!

Learn to own your actions, both good and bad. When you do something well, learn to accept praise for it. Learn to graciously say thank you and learn to celebrate yourself. When you make a mistake, learn to communicate and apologize for the error. Learn how to right the wrongs you can correct and also work to show yourself grace in areas where you miss the mark. Remind yourself that everyone makes mistakes, and work to move forward. Always celebrate yourself for taking responsibility for your actions too!

BARRIER #7: OVERCONFIDENCE

It's important to have an accurate assessment of your abilities. Be careful not to let your self-confidence slip beyond your sweet spot. Overconfidence looks like arrogance and complacency.

Overconfidence can destroy true self-confidence because it can sabotage and prevent you from presenting yourself in the best light at all times. For example, you may take on a project you cannot complete if you are overconfident. This can lead to disappointing people and make you feel embarrassed. These feelings of disappointment and embarrassment may cause your self-confidence to plummet.

How to remove this barrier: Be honest with yourself!

Learning to be aware of your abilities is being honest about your abilities and where they need growth. Stretching yourself is important, but knowing how far to stretch is even more important. Being realistic with what you know you can do versus what you wish you could do is key. It's not enough just to feel confident or to feel that level of belief in yourself. You have to do the work. You have to know who you are and what you can do. This takes time and must be a genuine and honest evaluation of yourself so that you can truly master the things that you're good at and truly become confident in yourself.

Brain Dump

Chapter 4

What barriers are getting in the way of your self-confidence?

_____

_____

_____

_____

_____

Notes, Thoughts, and Ideas

_____

_____

_____

_____

_____

Part 2

BECOMING A CEO
OF YOUR SELF-CONFIDENCE

"Believing in yourself and having confidence gives you outer strength."
— Nikki Bella

Chapter 5

CREATING
DAILY AFFIRMATIONS

id you know that your mind affects your actions more than any other part of your body? Your brain is powerful, and your brain controls the things you think, how your body moves, and the choices you make. Your brain is the most powerful organ in your body.

Most of the time, our brain is working to bring about positive change in our lives, but our brain is also working to keep us safe. This means that not only does our brain control our bodies, but it also controls our thoughts and our emotions. As a result, there are times when our brains work to prevent us from taking risks because it thinks we might experience danger.

Your thoughts play a major role in your overall wellness. The way you think and the way you move your thoughts are part of your mental health. It is our job to control our minds and our thoughts. When we control our thoughts and emotions, we feel more self-confident.

Affirmations are the small things we say to ourselves that help us improve the way we think.

They help us to stay in control of our thoughts, and they help us to ensure that our thoughts are focused on positive things rather than negativity. As you continue to develop your self-confidence, it is important to understand that becoming a person who truly believes in their abilities is someone who has taken control of their thoughts and works to ensure that their mindset and mental functioning are focused on belief statements rather than detrimental statements that cause their mindset or mental well-being to be negatively affected.

One of the ways that we can control our thoughts and keep our minds moving in the most positive directions is through affirmations. An affirmation is a concise yet powerful statement that allows you to be in control of your thoughts consciously. An affirmation is intentionally structured and carefully constructed so that the things you say have the most positive and powerful impact on your mindset.

When you say or think about them, affirmations become the thoughts that shape your reality; they become the thoughts that you believe about your situation, yourself, and abilities. Research has shown that around 80% of the subconscious thoughts you have in a day are negative ones. 80% of the things you think are critical are self-sabotaging thoughts.

Suppose you are to take control of your mind. You must be willing to stop comparing yourself with someone else and start looking internally at yourselves and working to ensure you are the healthiest and happiest you can be.

When we use affirmations, they make us consciously aware of our thoughts. So, when you consciously think positive thoughts, it's easier to control the negative ones, which always try to take over by making these positive declarations a part of your daily life. You are training your mind to prioritize positive thinking and not negative thinking. By making these affirmations every day, you are training your mind to believe in itself, in who you are, and in the value that you bring to the world.

Now, it's important to know how to write an affirmation so that it actually works. There are affirmations all over the place, many of which are wonderful. Some of them create a sense of hope or longing, but when trying to create new patterns and mindsets, we want to create present and true affirmations.

In this chapter, we will use 7 steps to help us write affirmations that will actually be effective and do the work we want them to do.

STEP 1: I AM

Beginning your affirmation with the words "I am" makes them powerful. "I am" or "I have" is a language that gives your subconscious mind command and makes it personal. In addition, "I am" makes your statement a "right now" statement rather than a statement of future wishing. When your mind hears the words "I am" or "I have," it takes the statement and interprets it as a directive that must be followed immediately.

STEP 2: BE PRESENT

When creating your affirmation, it is important to think about and say things as if they are happening in the present. Speaking in the present tense allows your mind to see things happening in the now. For example, you could say, "I will have a beautiful beach house one day," but your mind will see that as something to happen in the future and choose not to focus on making it happen because it isn't urgent. When you say, "I have a beautiful beach house," you allow your brain to visualize the house now and focus attention on making it a reality.

STEP 3: BE POSITIVE

Always speak about what you want and avoid speaking about what you don't want. Your affirmations should never use negatives. Instead of writing the affirmation "I never shut myself off to new opportunities," reword it to say "I am open to new opportunities."

STEP 4: KEEP IT SIMPLE

Your affirmations should always be short and concise. Don't write an essay; instead, make it easy to remember and state consistently and regularly.

STEP 5: BE SPECIFIC

Making specific affirmations allows your mind to visualize the outcome. It makes it easier to see exactly what you want to be or what you're describing. So instead of saying, "I will increase my income this year," say, "I am enjoying my hundred-thousand-dollar earnings this year.

STEP 6: MAKE IT PERSONAL

Always make sure that your affirmation describes your own actions. Do not use your affirmation to describe the actions of others or the actions you see in others. You may adopt an affirmation that applies to you, but do not write an affirmation that someone has told you to say. Write it for you.

STEP 7: MAKE IT MEANINGFUL

Make sure that your affirmation is important to you. Make sure it has meaning on all levels and speaks to you and who you are.

Brain Dump

Chapter 5

How important are affirmations to you?

_____

_____

_____

_____

_____

Notes, Thoughts, and Ideas

_____

_____

_____

_____

_____

Chapter 6

AFFIRMATIONS
YOU CAN USE

ffirmations are powerful, but only powerful when we use them correctly. So, it's important that you learn to identify powerful affirmations. It's important that you learn to write powerful affirmations, and it's important that you use them daily to change your mindset.

Affirmations allow you to become more self-confident. They will allow you to see yourself for who you truly are and to become more sure of your abilities, allowing you to be the CEO of your self-confidence.

This chapter is dedicated to well-written, strong, and powerful affirmations that you may use to begin the practice of making daily affirmations. As we discussed in Chapter 5, affirmations need to be personal and meaningful, so be sure to use only affirmations that feel good about who you truly are.

AFFIRMATIONS TO BUILD YOUR SELF-CONFIDENCE

I can say 'no'.

It's okay to say 'no'.

I have strong opinions, and my opinion counts.

I stand up for myself because it matters.

I stand up for myself because I matter.

I can achieve anything I set my mind to.

I am thankful for another day to grow, learn, and enjoy.

I embrace failure. Failure is feedback.

I accept the way I look without comparison.

I find ways to overcome my challenges.

I am always learning more about who I am and what matters to me.

I am excited when I get to change my mind.

It is okay for me to change my mind.

I ask for help when I need it.

I am beautiful.

Beauty comes in all shapes and sizes.

I am open to new possibilities.

I am excited by the challenge.

My dreams are achievable.

Today is my day.

Everything works out for the best.

I can take a break.

I listen to my body.

I make time for rest.

I matter.

I have a powerful voice.

Every problem has a solution.

I am starting now.

I am starting again.

I am fortunate.

Mistakes made yesterday are part of the beauty I am creating today.

When there's a bump in the road, I just keep going.

Today I am making progress.

Today, I am prepared.

I am prepared for success.

I am open to love.

I am open to happiness.

I am living in peace.

Joy is mine.

I am living in abundance.

I am the architect of my life.

I am blessed.

I am stronger than my challenges.

I am capable of attracting abundance.

I am a good friend.

I have good friends.

I believe in myself.

I am my best source of motivation.

I am achieving greatness.

I am capable of solving problems.

I attract joy and happiness.

I attract miracles.

I attract good friends.

I am creative.

I'm a powerful creator.

I'm surrounded by positive people.

I am surrounded by supportive people.

I am surrounded by people who believe in me.

I believe in myself

I take pride in my work.

I love myself unconditionally.

I am smart.

I am growing and changing for the better.

I love the person I am.

I love the person I am becoming.

I am becoming a better version of myself

I am strong.

I am powerful.

I am worthy.

I am wonderful.

I am wise.

I am confident in my personal choices.

My confidence is growing.

I am motivated.

I am positive.

I am confident in my abilities.

I'm confident in my skills.

I am confident in my gifts.

I radiate love.

I radiate self-confidence.

I am humble.

I am resilient.

I find solutions to my problems.

I am confident in my ability to change my life.

I have the tools and the resources to change my mind.

I have the resources to improve my life.

I am at peace.

I'm getting better every day and in every way.

I see the good in myself

I see the good in others.

I honor who I am.

I am proud of who I am.

I decide how I feel.

I am in charge of my thoughts.

Brain Dump

Chapter 6

Which affirmations feel most personal to you?

_____

_____

_____

_____

_____

Notes, Thoughts, and Ideas

_____

_____

_____

_____

_____

Chapter 7

WHAT IS YOUR SUPERPOWER?

I love superheroes. Their supernatural ability to take on villains, save the world, and restore good is exhilarating. As a fashion designer, I also love the ingenuity and beauty of their amazing super suits!

While I love superheroes and all they can do, I never fully understood what it meant when I heard teachers say that they had a superpower or what they were referring to when they would ask me about mine.

Have you ever wondered what it means to have a superpower? I am not a superhero. I can't scale skyscrapers like Spiderman or fly like Wonder Woman, and I will venture to guess that you can't either, but you do indeed have a superpower. We all do.

Your superpower is your contribution. It is the reason you were created, the role that you were put on this Earth to fill. It's what you do better than anyone else, and tapping into that power will not only help you live a meaningful life but will also help increase your self-confidence. Discovering your superpower will allow you to thrive at school, at work, and in every aspect of your life.

> Superpower = The unique, exceptional ability that allows you to fulfill the purpose for which you were created.

For years, I wondered what my superpower was. I knew that I was good at organizing and designing. I enjoy being creative and making friends, but none of those really seemed to be a superpower. None of those felt like an exceptional ability that made me stand out.

During my sophomore year of high school, my mom encouraged me to apply for a Leadership Douglas program. The mission of Leadership Douglas is to identify, encourage, and develop leadership abilities so that its participants grow personally and professionally. It was an honor to be selected. However, I wasn't really sure how the program would help me. At the time, I didn't consider myself a leader and certainly didn't think leadership was something unique. I just assumed anyone could be a leader, but it was during this 10-week experience that I discovered that leadership itself is a superpower.

Not everyone has the strength or the ability to lead people. It requires exceptional skills to effectively listen to people and guide them toward a common goal. I've discovered that my superpower is leadership.

This is exciting because as I discover my superpower, I can more confidently step into situations requiring a person with great leadership skills. I have the self-confidence to say "Yes" in situations in which I might normally have been hesitant or nervous.

This is why it is important, as the CEO of your self-confidence, to identify your exceptional skills, your major strengths, and those areas where you truly stand out. This will allow you to become more self-confident in your unique, extraordinary abilities, and it will allow you to seek out opportunities where you can shine your brightest.

So how do you discover your superpower?

There are lots of things that you can do to identify your superpower. For instance, I found my superpower when I attended a program geared toward my strengths, but I attended that program because my mother saw something in me. People will often see something in you that you don't readily see in yourself.

In this chapter, you will spend time reflecting on and answering a series of questions. I encourage you to find a quiet space and take your time answering these questions. Ask people you trust to help you with any questions you have difficulty answering. Once you've responded to each question, review them for any patterns. Those patterns will reveal your super powers and give you a place on which to focus and develop.

1. What comes naturally to you?

2. What feels effortless when you are doing it?

3. How do you amaze others?

4. What makes you willing to sacrifice your time and effort?

5. What areas do you find yourself in where you are fearless?

6. What can you see more clearly than others?

7. What fills you with passion?

8. What makes time disappear?

9. What makes you different from others?

10. What advice do your friends ask you for often?

11. What do friends always ask you to help them with?

12. What makes you happiest?

13. What do you love to do that your parents, teachers, or friends might overlook or ignore because you do it so effortlessly and so quickly?

14. What do you do effortlessly that you think everyone can do easily?

Getting clarity about your strengths can make all the difference in your life, schoolwork, and the future; the number one thing you can do is identify your strengths and your superpower. Look over the answers that you provided to the questions above. Do you see patterns? Is there something that seems to be consistently repeated that you never realized? This is probably your superpower.

Now, as the CEO of your self-confidence, I want you to begin thinking about how you can nurture this superpower.

What opportunities can you say "Yes" to?

What training, classes, or workshops are available to develop this superpower?

As you begin developing your superpower, your self-confidence will also get stronger because you'll know exactly what things you can tackle and accomplish well.

Brain Dump

Chapter 7

What is your superpower? How do you know?

_____

_____

_____

_____

_____

Notes, Thoughts, and Ideas

_____

_____

_____

_____

_____

Chapter 8

TAKE A QUIZ, DISCOVER YOUR STRENGTHS

*I*n Chapter 7, we talked about discovering your superpower. In that chapter, you answered a series of questions that would allow you to identify patterns within yourself that could help uncover your superpower. Your special, one-of-a-kind skills and abilities set you apart from other people and help you do what you are made to do.

Those patterns emerged quickly, clearly, and easily for some of you. For others, identifying patterns may have been a struggle. Either way, this chapter will provide you with additional tools to help you identify your strengths and continue to develop your self-confidence.

This chapter is dedicated to discovering your strengths through personality tests. A personality test is a tool used to help you better understand yourself and your personality in relation to other people. These tests are used to explore how your differences compare to aspects of other people's lives.

Reflecting and answering truthfully without hesitation is the best way to answer these questions and better understand yourself. There are no right or wrong answers to the questions on these tests, and the information you gather can be used to clarify who you are and where you might best thrive when it comes to school, work, and play. These tests are helpful because they provide you with an overview of your strengths and weaknesses; they help you to identify the paths that you can take to achieve success in your life, and they help you build and strengthen relationships because they provide a way to help you understand the things you like and the things you dislike. They are great tools that can help you express yourself more authentically.

I will share 6 of the best personality tests specifically geared toward teens and young adults. All of the tests in this chapter are free to use and may be accessed in many places across the internet. Each can be completed using the notes pages in the book, on your phone or tablet, or they may also be printed.

In order to access these personality tests, scan the QR code with your camera phone or tablet, and you will be taken directly to the personality test being highlighted. You may also access each assessment using the web address listed in the reference section. I've also included brief descriptions of the personalities derived from each test.

1. PERSONALITY TEST FOR TEENS

This test aims to develop the traits related to your emotional intelligence, like empathy, motivation, and consciousness. It is based on the Jungian Mental Mechanisms created by Carl Gustav Jung.

This personality quiz is specifically for young people 13 years of age and older. It has 20 questions that assess your preferences and your style. The personality types are divided into four categories: extraversion/introversion, planned/spontaneous, hands-on/theoretical, and objective/subjective.

2. 5-MINUTE PERSONALITY TEST

This particular personality test was developed by comparing your results with four animal categories:

Lions, Otters, Golden Retrievers, and beavers. The test claims that we are all a combination of these four animal characteristics, but the two animals with the highest scores will reveal your personality. Each animal has its own strengths and weaknesses, and a list containing these traits is provided at the end of the test. There are only ten questions, so this personality quiz is easy and quick to complete.

3. THE BIG FIVE PERSONALITY TEST

This test is very simple. It helps you discover which letter you are in the ocean. OCEAN is an acronym for openness, conscientiousness, extraversion,

agreeableness, and neuroticism. This is one of the most widely used personality tests, so you can find a lot of information on this test.

4. THE HOLLAND CODE TEST

This is a commonly used test given during job interviews and career counseling, and it's most suitable for high school students who are about to enter college or begin thinking about their careers.

Six categories represent the different personality types: realistic, investigative, artistic, socially enterprising, and conventional.

Completing this test is also pretty simple. You just have to read the scenarios and decide which one relates to you the most. Then you will tally up your scores. When you are finished, you will discover which personality type you have, and which career path will most likely make you happy and successful as you develop your skills.

5. THE TRUE COLORS PERSONALITY TEST

The True Colors personality test is one of the most popular personality tests out there. It was created using the colors blue, orange, gold, and green to categorize the strengths of young people and students. When you take this test, you will be given a series of questions that will help you rate your preferences. You can either have one primary color to represent you, or you can be a combination of this test. It works to help you and the people around you understand your innermost thoughts and your desires.

While these tests are subjective and the results are not scientific facts, they can be very insightful. Understanding your personality type is a good way of understanding yourself better. These tests can help you understand your behaviors and what you need to develop and grow. Knowing your personality type can also help you develop your self-confidence.

Use the QR codes to begin. A brief description of the results can be found on the following pages. Have fun with these personality tests and record your responses on the organizer found on the next page to see if any patterns emerge.

UNDERSTANDING YOUR RESULTS

PERSONALITY TEST FOR TEENS

Mover Personality Style (Hands-on and spontaneous)
Core Value: Freedom

The Mover personality is courageous, exploratory, and playful. Movers seek action and adventure. They crave variety and enjoy improvising. Movers are good at thinking on their feet. They automatically find the fastest way to do things and make them fun. They change course as often as needed and aren't likely to let bumps in the road slow them down.

Connector Personality Style (Theoretical and Subjective)
Core Value: Relationship

The connector personality type is considerate, cooperative, and encouraging. Connectors seek harmony and personal connection.

They prefer to make decisions that feel good and are in alignment with their values. Connectors naturally interact with others and connect meaning to events. They excel at recognizing strength in others and place high importance on personal growth.

Thinker Personality Style (Theoretical and objective)
Core Value: Competency

The Thinker Personality style is curious, logical, and self-sufficient. Thinkers seek clarity and knowledge. They prefer to make calculated decisions. Thinkers explore all aspects of an issue and can't help but suggest new ways of doing things. They need time to think before making decisions. They can be fiercely independent and value their privacy.

Planner Personality Style (Hands-On and Planned)
Core Value: Responsibility

The Planner personality style is organized, prepared, and dependable. Planners seek order and fairness. They crave consistency and have things in their place. Planners are naturally able to distinguish right from wrong. They like to keep their personal space well-tended and pay attention to details. They seek a sense of completion and enjoy crossing items off a list.

ANIMAL PERSONALITY TEST

L= Lions

Lions are leaders. They are usually the bosses at work (or at least they think they are). They are decisive, bottom-line folks who are observers, not watchers or listeners. They love to solve problems. They are usually individualists and love to seek new adventures and opportunities. Lions are very confident and self-reliant. In a group setting, if no one else takes charge, the lion will. Unfortunately, if they don't learn how to tone down their aggressiveness, their natural dominating traits can cause problems with others. Most entrepreneurs are strong lions, or at least have a lot of lions in them.

O= Otters

Otters are excitable, fun-seeking cheerleader types who love to talk. They're great at motivating others, and they need to be in an environment where they can talk and have a vote on major decisions. The Otter's outgoing nature makes them great networkers. They usually know a lot of people who know a lot of people. They can be very loving and encouraging, unless under pressure. They strongly desire to be liked and enjoy being the center of attention. They are often very attentive to style, clothes, and flash. Otters are the life of any party; most people enjoy being around them.

G= Golden retrievers

One word describes these people: loyal. They are so loyal that they can absorb the most emotional pain and punishment in a relationship and stay committed. They are great listeners, incredibly empathetic, and warm-hearted encouragers. However, they tend to be such people-pleasers that they can have great difficulty asserting themselves in a situation or relationship when needed.

B= Beavers

Beavers have a strong need to do things right and by the book. They are the kind of people who actually read instructional manuals. They are great at providing quality control in an office. They will provide quality control in any situation or field that demands accuracy, such as accounting or engineering, because rules, consistency, and high standards are so important to Beavers. They are often frustrated with others who do not share these same characteristics. Their strong need to maintain high and often unrealistic standards can short-circuit their ability to express warmth in a relationship.

THE BIG FIVE PERSONALITY TEST

(O) **Openness to experience** is the personality trait of seeking new experiences and intellectual pursuits. High scorers may daydream a lot, and low scorers may be very down-to-earth.

(C) **Conscientiousness** is the personality trait of being honest and hard-working. High scorers tend to follow the rules and prefer clean homes. Low scorers may be messy.

(E) **Extraversion** is the personality trait of seeking fulfillment from sources outside of oneself or in the community. High scorers tend to be very social, while low scorers prefer to work on projects alone.

(A) **Agreeableness** influences how people adjust their behavior to accommodate others. Low scorers tend to tell it like it is.

(N) **Neuroticism** is the personality trait of being emotional.

THE HOLLAND CODE PERSONALITY TEST

R= Realistic

These people are often good at mechanical or athletic jobs. Good college majors and careers for realistic people are:

- Agriculture
- Health assistant
- Computers
- Construction
- Mechanics
- Engineering
- Food and Hospitality

I= Investigative

These people like to watch, learn, analyze, and solve problems. Good college majors and careers for investigative people are:

- Marine Biology
- Engineering
- Chemistry
- Zoology
- Medicine
- Consumer Economics
- Psychology

A= Artistic

These people like to work in an unstructured situation where they can use their creativity. Good majors and careers for artistic people are:

- Communications

- Cosmetology
- Fine and Performing Arts
- Photography
- Radio and TV.
- Interior Design
- Architecture

S= Social

These people like to work with other people rather than things. Good college majors and careers for social people are:

- Counseling
- Nursing
- Physical Therapy
- T ravel
- Advertising
- Public Relations
- Education

E= Enterprising

These people like to work with others and enjoy persuading and performing. Good college majors and careers for enterprising people are:

- Fashion Merchandising
- Real Estate
- Marketing/Sales
- Law
- Political Science
- International Trade
- Banking/Finance

C= Conventional

These people are very detail-oriented, organized, and like to work with data. Good college majors and careers for conventional people are:

- Accounting
- Court Reporting
- Insurance
- Administration
- Medical Records
- Banking
- Data Processing

THE TRUE COLORS PERSONALITY TEST

Blue

Relationship-Oriented, Caretaker

The "BLUE" personality type thrives the most in relationships and gauging the feelings of others. They are typically quiet, social, and compassionate, always seeking the group's good. They will also be the first to reach out to those that may be struggling or hurting and can be counted on for support in tough times.

Green

Cognitively Oriented, Intellectually Independent

The "GREEN" personality type is highly analytical. They can quickly see patterns in nearly anything and thrive on accumulating the most information possible before making a decision. They are always ready to learn something new and enjoy the challenge of learning. Their focus may wander at times, but they are constantly taking in as much stimulus as possible. This can sometimes wear them out, so time to recharge and refresh their minds is vital. As for their money, they invest it.

Gold

Structure Oriented, Natural Leader

The "GOLD" personality type is a natural leader. They are serious, hardworking, and highly emphasize quality, organization, accuracy, and decisive action. They respect those that show respect and always want to be seen as dependable and trustworthy. Their actions are planned to the letter, and they do not have time or patience for unexpected complications. They show they care by their actions for their loved ones as well as for their money. They are good at saving it.

Orange

Adventurous Action Taker

The "ORANGE" personality type often has overwhelming energy and is comfortable taking action without being overly analytical about the optimal direction. They are more inclined to use their gut instinct to choose a more risk-laden path over a safe option and may reap great rewards for their boldness and decisiveness. Oranges need to feel as if they are in control of themselves and their situation. They typically resist being confined and weighed down by too many calendar commitments or needy people in relationships. As for their money, they spend it.

Discover your Strengths

Take time to complete each of the personality tests included in this chapter.
Capture your results here and look for any patterns.

Pesonality Test for Teens Top Style:	Animal Personality Test Top Animal:
Big Five Personality Test Top Trait:	True Colors Personality Test Core Color:

Holland Code Test
Interest Code

- - - - - - - - - -   - - - - - - - - - -   - - - - - - - - - -

Brain Dump

Chapter 8

What are your greatest strengths?

_____

_____

_____

_____

_____

Notes, Thoughts, and Ideas

_____

_____

_____

_____

_____

Chapter 9

JOURNALING IS LIT!

While it is true that I discovered my leadership superpower while in high school, I have been developing my self-confidence for years. In fact, my parents began very early, assisting me in understanding and strengthening my unique abilities. My parents have always encouraged me to trust myself by teaching me strategies for reflection and routines.

When I was 7 years old, my mom gave me my first journal. I didn't know it then, but this was the beginning of my self-confidence work. My journal was the place where I captured all of my craziest stories, confided my saddest moments, and shared my deepest thoughts. My journal allowed me to be heard when I didn't want to speak out loud.

Research has shown that journaling is one of the most powerful self-confidence-building activities you can do. That's right, more powerful than affirmations, working out, drinking water, or taking good care of yourself, even though those are very important.

And journaling is simple.

If you learn how to journal and do it consistently, it can transform and improve your self-confidence, mental health, emotional health, and even physical health.

Journaling is basically a way for you to write down your thoughts and feelings as you reflect and think about your everyday life. Journaling gives you a place to express gratitude, which stimulates positive emotions. Journaling helps you work through challenges and can help you heal from past wounds and decrease stress. Journaling builds resiliency, one of the most important skills for success and growth.

The wonderful thing about journaling is that there's no right or wrong way to do it. It's something that is very personal and can come in many forms.

I know people who keep a journal on their phones by recording voice memos. Other people keep a journal by doing brain dumps at the end of the day. Another way is to write in a traditional diary. Some people journal by keeping a list of the things they want to remember or a list of goals they want to accomplish. While others keep a journal by writing down all their blessings or answered prayers. My journaling is a combination of all of these.

The real power of journaling comes from developing a habit of journaling and doing it consistently. This means journaling every day, not just when you're experiencing stress or anxiety.

The best way to get started with journaling is to START. Remind yourself that your journal is for your eyes only. You don't have to have good spelling. You don't have to have great punctuation. It doesn't even have to make sense because your journal is for your old eyes only. Allow your journal to be a safe and judgment-free space.

Create a writing routine. Creating a time every single day where you have blocked off time to journal, whether for 10 minutes, 20 minutes, or 5 minutes, will force you to stop and actually do the work of building your self-confidence.

Don't limit yourself to only one way of journaling. Find a journaling technique that works for you. There are many different techniques; the best part is that you can use as many as you want. The goal is to get your thoughts out and to be consistent.

Here are a few of the techniques I have used in the past, along with tips on how you may have the most success using them.

FREE WRITING

The free writing technique is used to allow space for your mind to flow freely. You could also think of this as brain dumping or brainstorming. You spend the entire time writing by setting a timer or creating the goal of filling a specified number of pages. If you run out of ideas, you just keep writing, whatever comes to your mind. Free writing is incredibly powerful. It helps you to unpack confusing situations or make sense of mixed emotions. Free writing is about getting things out and not making them sound perfect or polished.

Tips on using the free-writing technique:

- Start small. Begin with 5-10 minutes at a time and gradually increase your time.

- Start by describing your feelings, your surroundings, or things that bother you.

LISTS

Lists are a great way to write when you find free writing a little too challenging. Lists are an incredible journaling technique that can help you organize, keep track of, and record anything you want to remember related to school, family, work, or life in general. Lists can be quicker than doing a big journal page and might feel less intimidating than other journaling techniques.

Tips on using the list technique:

- Keep a running list of your favorite books, movies, recipes, or places you'd like to visit.

- Start a new list each day and reflect on it at the end of the day.

ART JOURNALING

If you like capturing your ideas or thoughts through pictures, you should try creating an art journal. An art journal is a great place for sketches and doodles. There aren't any rules when keeping an art journal, and there's no one right way to do it. You can always mix different ideas and images to really help bring out your thoughts and ideas. It's the best way for you to explore your creativity, keep track of your ideas, and work through challenges.

Tips for using an Art Journal:

- Think outside of the box.

- Begin by illustrating feelings in multiple ways.

- Create without judgment, remembering that your journal is for your eyes only.

THE UNSENT LETTER

Using this technique of writing an unsent letter is a way for you to share your thoughts without feeling like someone will see them. It gives you a great way to forgive someone who might have hurt you or to gain peace of mind about a situation that you might not be able to resolve any other way than through a letter. Whether it's by expressing your feelings to an ex-boyfriend or someone who may have passed away, writing a letter can give voice to everything you want to say.

Tips for using an unsent letter:

- Only write for your eyes.

- Write different types of letters. Letters of gratitude, forgiveness, and letters to share exciting, scary, or intimidating news.

BULLET JOURNALS

Instead of blank, lined pages, a bullet journal contains sections for daily things to do, calendars, notes, and goals. It is a great way to get organized by keeping track of your reminders and schedules and having them all in one place.

Tips for using a bullet journal:

- A bullet journal isn't something you buy already templated. Instead, you purchase a blank or dot grid notebook and create something unique to you and your goals.
- Always include an index and a calendar.
- Enjoy the process of designing your perfect journal.

THREE THINGS JOURNAL

A three-things journal helps you to gain perspective on your day. It can help you think about and plan out your day, and it can also help you keep track of your goals. Each day you write down three goals you're working toward, three things you're letting go of, and three things you're grateful for. This short exercise helps you focus on your priorities, infuse positivity into your day and let go of negative emotions or anxieties.

READING JOURNAL

A reading journal is a place for you to keep track of your thoughts related to anything you read. Whether it is an article, books, magazines, or blogs, a reading journal helps you get more from those experiences.

Tips for using a reading journal:

- Keep track of the books you read.

- While reading, think about and write down the lessons learned from the books you are reading.

- You may also use this technique to agree or disagree with the books you read.

PROMPT JOURNALING

A prompt journal is a journal that provides you with prompts or sentence starters. These prompts are a great way to get you thinking and allow you to create a writing routine.

Tips for using a prompt journal:

- Find prompts that work for you.

- Don't limit yourself to the few lines provided. If a prompt leads you to deeper thought, be sure to capture all of your thoughts regarding that idea.

With these powerful journaling techniques and ideas, you now have everything you need to get started. Remember, there is no right or wrong way to journal, so try one or all of the techniques mentioned in this chapter and find the journal that works best for you.

Journaling is one of the best ways to start building your self-confidence. As the CEO of your self-confidence, it's your responsibility to begin taking seriously the act of organizing your thoughts and processing them so that you can continue to grow and become the person who really truly believes in yourself and knows how they shine best.

Brain Dump

Chapter 9

What type of journaling would you like to try? Why?

_____

_____

_____

_____

_____

**Notes, Thoughts,
and Ideas**

_____

_____

_____

_____

_____

Chapter 10

GETTING ORGANIZED

I love success! I have always loved getting good grades, learning new things, and the feeling of doing well in my classes and accomplishing my goals. When I was in elementary school, success and getting good grades were easy. All my work was kept on a desk with my name on it. Teachers would remind us of upcoming assignments, and my parents reviewed my homework every day at the end of the night.

When I got to middle school, things became a little more challenging, and keeping track of things was a struggle. I remember very specifically a project I had to complete. I had a plan in my mind of what I wanted to do and how I wanted it to be done, but there were so many other things on my plate as well. I was in volleyball, musical theater, a part of student government, and active in the church. With all I had going on, the work of completing my assignment just kept getting overlooked.

The night before the assignment was due, I popped up from the couch, ran into my mom's room, and begged her to help me get it done. My mom was unhappy, and while I wish I could say she ran me to the store and helped me get it done, that is not the case. I missed the deadline and, as a result, did not get the desired grade.

This experience taught me a very important lesson: if I were going to continue to be successful, I would have to get organized. My mom and dad were a great help. They helped me develop the organizational skills I have today, which were a crucial part of growing my self-confidence.

As the CEO of your self-confidence, it is important that you understand just how important organization is to building a healthy self-confidence. I believe that the environment you create for yourself directly connects to your capacity to think clearly. Being organized gives you a sense of control in your life. You control how your day begins and progresses, what tasks you complete and accomplish, and where and when things will take place. Having control over your life is so important to feeling confident in yourself because you feel so much more grounded, which keeps the anxiety of wondering whether or not you forgot something from consuming your thoughts.

Over the years, I have learned that you can do a couple of things to help you become a more organized person. If you have already mastered your organizational skills, perhaps some of the things I share in this chapter will help you improve on your current system. If you struggle with being organized, these simple strategies will help you become more organized and self-confident

4 KEYS TO ORGANIZING YOUR LIFE:

KEY #1 GIVE EVERYTHING A PLACE

Have you ever been ready to walk out the door on time and realized you don't have the phone or iPad you need for class? You spend the next 15 minutes rushing around the house looking for it, and when you finally find it in your sock drawer, you discover that you are now late for school. This is so frustrating and can have a significant impact on your self-confidence. So one way to minimize these experiences is to dedicate a space for your things. Put your backpack in the same place every day, hang your keys on their hook, and use your creative juices to repurpose something or create something to hold your air pods, chargers, and other important items. Putting things in a specified spot makes finding them easy and allows your mind to focus on other, more important things.

KEY #2 DECLUTTER DAILY

Empty your purse, backpack, and sports bag every day. Throw away garbage and organize important papers. Use this time to look through assignments and paperwork that needs parental attention. Look through everything in your bag and put items in their specified place. Take care of any tasks that need to be taken care of right then while they are fresh. Don't put them off until later; if you must, be sure to add them to your list of tasks to be completed.

KEY #3 CREATE AND FOLLOW DAILY ROUTINES

I've said this a few times throughout this book, but one of the best ways to build self-confidence is to follow a routine. A routine is simply the sequence of actions you perform the same way every time. A schedule is a type of routine, especially as a student, and creating a schedule or routine is a great way to build organizational skills.

Make a strategy for completing the task at hand. Assign days and times and stick to the plan. Develop a morning, after school, and bedtime routine. Some of the things you should have in your routine to really boost your self-confidence include:

<u>Morning Routine</u>

- Daily affirmation/prayer/meditation
- Make your bed
- Morning Hygiene
- Breakfast

<u>After School Routine</u>

- Empty Bags
- Put things where they belong
- Add tasks to the planner/calendar/to-do list
- Homework
- Relax

Bedtime Routine

- Select an outfit for the following day

- Pack bags and place them at the door

- Tidy desk and bedroom

- Evening Hygiene

- Evening reflection/journaling/meditation

Always create a general plan and stick to it for at least 90 days. After 90 days, reflect on the plan. Consider the things that worked along with the things that did not and adjust where necessary.

KEY #4 USE ORGANIZATIONAL TOOLS

Organizational tools such as calendars, planners, notepads, and whiteboards are great for organizing. I think everyone should have a strategy for planning out their days and weeks. Planners are the best way to do this, and while finding the planner that works best for you, finding one that allows you to see all of your tasks in one place is best.

Carrying a notepad or using the voice memo app on your phone to capture thoughts or reminders can help you remember tasks that pop up throughout the day, and having a whiteboard hung on your bedroom wall can help you keep track of routines and schedules.

Becoming more organized brings many benefits, including greater self-confidence, better performance, and improved mental health. Taking steps to organize your day will help you start quickly, find everything you need, and focus effectively to complete your daily tasks. Take time to find the tools to help you feel organized and in control.

Brain Dump

Chapter 10

In what part of your life could you be more organized?

_____

_____

_____

_____

Notes, Thoughts, and Ideas

_____

_____

_____

_____

Chapter 11

THE PERFECT PLANNER

As a young CEO and business owner, my life is pretty busy. In addition to being a fashion designer and boutique owner. I am also a certified public speaker. I maintain a high academic GPA, serve as the president of my high school's National Honor Society and Future Business Leaders of America chapter, and am highly involved in church and community service. I don't have a lot of spare time, but in my spare time, I love shopping, upcycling, and snuggling with my pet Yorkie, Sweetie Coco Cake.

So, as you can see, I am a pretty busy girl and don't have much time. The only way I can be successful and maintain my busy life is by ensuring that I am organized and planning out my days well.

In chapter 10, we talked about being organized and the tools that can be used for planning. In this chapter, I want to talk to you about the art of planning and how you can find the perfect planner for you.

While I'm not going to say that a planner is right for everyone, I will definitely say that planners are the most useful and most effective way to become organized. As we learned in chapter 10, being organized is a major key to becoming the CEO of your self-confidence.

We all have very different lives and very different needs. This is why there's not one single organizer or planning system that will work for everyone. It's also true that planners are not magical; the only way they work is if you use them. So it's most important to pick a planner that meets your needs right now.

With so many planner options on the market, how can you choose the best one for you? There are a few things to keep in mind when searching for your perfect planner, but before we jump into this wonderful world of planners, there is something you should keep in mind. Finding your perfect planner is all about being open to experiment and exploration. So be prepared to try many different planners. If you don't love it, keep track of the reasons for your dislike and then switch it up. Keep looking, don't give up.

Now let's find your perfect planner!

Many paper planners are out there, and they can range in style. I personally prefer paper planners over digital ones, but if you are more of a minimalist or technology lover, you might prefer using a digital planner app. Digital planners are portable and can be set to give audible notifications; if a digital planner sounds like more of your style, do some research to find the planner that will work best for you.

The following information will focus specifically on paper planners, but many of the ideas will also give you something to think about when choosing a digital planner.

LAYOUT

You want to make sure that when choosing the layout for your planner, you consider your lifestyle. Will you need a monthly, weekly, or daily layout? If you like to plan your days hour by hour, a daily planner with an hourly layout would probably be the best choice.

If you are in high school or college, you probably have a consistent schedule where most of your hours are spent in classes. Using a daily or hourly layout wouldn't be as helpful to you because large sections of your planner might go unused. A weekly layout is a great option for students who like to see the entire week in front of them. Planners with a weekly layout also provide spaces where you can write down all the tasks that must be done throughout the week.

Monthly planners are great if you like simplicity and you're not a big list maker. If you just need to know where you should be on specific day or if you want to remember birthdays and major appointments or major events a monthly view layout would be best for you.

SIZE

Pick a planner size that is comfortable for you. Regarding planners, size is important because the planner's size and weight will determine how often you carry it around, and planners are most effective when you have them right at your fingertips.

A pocket planner is a great way for you to take notes. It's small and it's for people who don't have a lot of things to keep track of.

Small to medium planners are portable and can easily fit in your backpack or your purse. They are great for keeping track of schedules and tasks and for jotting down notes or ideas.

A large planner will take up more space. They are heavier to carry around, so you might just find yourself leaving them on a desk. This is not the best type of planner for students or people on the go. However, if you use your planner to see the month or daily schedule at a glance, a large planner might be appropriate.

STYLE

What is your planning style? While there's no right or wrong style, it's important for you to know the kind of planner you are. If you are creative and crafty and like to have planners that look really beautiful, then you might want to have a planner with lots of room for sketching, journaling, and doodling.

If you are more of a logical thinker and like to plan more logically, you might not need all of the stickers and cutesy things that come from those more creative planners.

BINDING

The binding of your planner describes the way the pages stay together. Spiral-bound planners are pretty popular, and one of the best things about these types of planners is that they can lie flat. Softbound and hardcover planners are less bulky and easier to carry around because they aren't easily bent up or destroyed.

Refillable ring or disc-bound planners allow you to add and remove pages easily without the mess you would get with a spiral-bound planner. These planners also offer a bit more versatility and personalization.

Now it's time to begin thinking about what you need in a planner. Everyone's needs are different, and ultimately, a planner is a personal preference. Take time to do your research, but don't overthink it. You can always change your mind; there is nothing wrong with trying something new. The fun is in the discovery, so get started today. It's time to find your perfect planner.

Brain Dump

Chapter 11

What type of planner do you think is best for you? Why?

_____

_____

_____

_____

_____

**Notes, Thoughts,
and Ideas**

_____

_____

_____

_____

_____

Part 3

PUTTING IT
ALL TOGETHER

"Optimism is the faith that leads to achievement. Nothing can be done without hope and confidence."
– Helen Keller

Chapter 12

MY AFFIRMATIONS

Use this space to create your own daily affirmations.
Remember they should be present tense, positive,
simple, specific, personal, and meaningful.

Daily AFFIRMATIONS

REMEMBER...

- ☑ PRESENT
- ☑ POSITIVE
- ☑ SIMPLE

- ☑ SPECIFIC
- ☑ PERSONAL
- ☑ MEANINGFUL

I AM...

I HAVE...

EVERYTHING IS...

Daily AFFIRMATIONS

REMEMBER...

- ☑ PRESENT
- ☑ POSITIVE
- ☑ SIMPLE

- ☑ SPECIFIC
- ☑ PERSONAL
- ☑ MEANINGFUL

Daily AFFIRMATIONS

REMEMBER...

- ☑ PRESENT
- ☑ POSITIVE
- ☑ SIMPLE

- ☑ SPECIFIC
- ☑ PERSONAL
- ☑ MEANINGFUL

Daily AFFIRMATIONS

REMEMBER...

- ☑ PRESENT
- ☑ POSITIVE
- ☑ SIMPLE

- ☑ SPECIFIC
- ☑ PERSONAL
- ☑ MEANINGFUL

Daily AFFIRMATIONS

REMEMBER...

- ✓ PRESENT
- ✓ POSITIVE
- ✓ SIMPLE

- ✓ SPECIFIC
- ✓ PERSONAL
- ✓ MEANINGFUL

Daily AFFIRMATIONS

REMEMBER...

- ☑ PRESENT
- ☑ POSITIVE
- ☑ SIMPLE

- ☑ SPECIFIC
- ☑ PERSONAL
- ☑ MEANINGFUL

Chapter 13

MY JOURNAL

Start journaling today,
use this area to get in the zone!

Daily Journal

Date_____

Daily Affirmation

Dump zone for ideas...

Today I am grateful for...

1._____
_____
2._____
_____
3._____
_____

My To-Do list for the day...

1._____
_____
2._____
_____
3._____
_____

Thoughts about my day...

☐ Drank Water
☐ Meditated/Quiet Time
☐ Exercised

☐ Act of Kindness
☐ Finished homework
☐ Had fun

Daily Journal

Date_____

Daily Affirmation

Dump zone for ideas...

Today I am grateful for...

1._____
_____
2._____
_____
3._____
_____

Thoughts about my day...

My To-Do list for the day...

1._____
_____
2._____
_____
3._____
_____

☐ Drank Water
☐ Meditated/Quiet Time
☐ Exercised

☐ Act of Kindness
☐ Finished homework
☐ Had fun

Daily Journal

Date_____

Daily Affirmation

Dump zone for ideas...

Today I am grateful for...

1._____
_____
2._____
_____
3._____
_____

Thoughts about my day...

My To-Do list for the day...

1._____
_____
2._____
_____
3._____
_____

☐ Drank Water
☐ Meditated/Quiet Time
☐ Exercised

☐ Act of Kindness
☐ Finished homework
☐ Had fun

Daily Journal

Date_____

Daily Affirmation

Dump zone for ideas...

Today I am grateful for...

1._____
_____
2._____
_____
3._____
_____

My To-Do list for the day...

1._____
_____
2._____
_____
3._____
_____

Thoughts about my day...

☐ Drank Water
☐ Meditated/Quiet Time
☐ Exercised

☐ Act of Kindness
☐ Finished homework
☐ Had fun

Daily Journal

Date_____

Daily Affirmation

Dump zone for ideas...

Today I am grateful for...

1._____

_____

2._____

_____

3._____

_____

My To-Do list for the day...

1._____

_____

2._____

_____

3._____

_____

Thoughts about my day...

☐ Drank Water
☐ Meditated/Quiet Time
☐ Exercised

☐ Act of Kindness
☐ Finished homework
☐ Had fun

Daily Journal

Date_____

Daily Affirmation

Dump zone for ideas...

Today I am grateful for...

1._____

_____

2._____

_____

3._____

_____

My To-Do list for the day...

1._____

_____

2._____

_____

3._____

_____

Thoughts about my day...

☐ Drank Water
☐ Meditated/Quiet Time
☐ Exercised

☐ Act of Kindness
☐ Finished homework
☐ Had fun

Daily Journal

Date_____

Daily Affirmation

Dump zone for ideas...

Today I am grateful for...

1._____
_____
2._____
_____
3._____
_____

Thoughts about my day...

My To-Do list for the day...

1._____
_____
2._____
_____
3._____
_____

☐ Drank Water
☐ Meditated/Quiet Time
☐ Exercised

☐ Act of Kindness
☐ Finished homework
☐ Had fun

Daily Journal

Date_____

Daily Affirmation

Dump zone for ideas...

Today I am grateful for...

1._____
_____
2._____
_____
3._____
_____

Thoughts about my day...

My To-Do list for the day...

1._____
_____
2._____
_____
3._____
_____

☐ Drank Water
☐ Meditated/Quiet Time
☐ Exercised

☐ Act of Kindness
☐ Finished homework
☐ Had fun

Daily Journal

Date_____

Daily Affirmation

Dump zone for ideas...

Today I am grateful for...

1._____

_____

2._____

_____

3._____

_____

My To-Do list for the day...

1._____

_____

2._____

_____

3._____

_____

Thoughts about my day...

☐ Drank Water
☐ Meditated/Quiet Time
☐ Exercised

☐ Act of Kindness
☐ Finished homework
☐ Had fun

Daily Journal

Date_____

Daily Affirmation

Dump zone for ideas...

Today I am grateful for...

1._____

_____

2._____

_____

3._____

_____

Thoughts about my day...

My To-Do list for the day...

1._____

_____

2._____

_____

3._____

_____

☐ Drank Water
☐ Meditated/Quiet Time
☐ Exercised

☐ Act of Kindness
☐ Finished homework
☐ Had fun

Daily Journal

Date_____

Daily Affirmation

Dump zone for ideas...

Today I am grateful for...

1._____
_____
2._____
_____
3._____
_____

My To-Do list for the day...

1._____
_____
2._____
_____
3._____
_____

Thoughts about my day...

☐ Drank Water
☐ Meditated/Quiet Time
☐ Exercised

☐ Act of Kindness
☐ Finished homework
☐ Had fun

Daily Journal

Date_____

Daily Affirmation

Dump zone for ideas...

Today I am grateful for...

1._____
_____
2._____
_____
3._____
_____

Thoughts about my day...

My To-Do list for the day...

1._____
_____
2._____
_____
3._____
_____

☐ Drank Water
☐ Meditated/Quiet Time
☐ Exercised

☐ Act of Kindness
☐ Finished homework
☐ Had fun

Daily Journal

Date_____

Daily Affirmation

Dump zone for ideas...

Today I am grateful for...

1._____
_____
2._____
_____
3._____
_____

My To-Do list for the day...

1._____
_____
2._____
_____
3._____
_____

Thoughts about my day...

☐ Drank Water
☐ Meditated/Quiet Time
☐ Exercised

☐ Act of Kindness
☐ Finished homework
☐ Had fun

Chapter 14

MY CHECKLIST

Use this checklist to ensure you have

everything you need to become

the CEO of your self-confidence.

Everything I need as CEO of my Self-Confidence

☐ An understanding of what self-confidence is and is not.

☐ Time and space for daily reflection.

☐ Systems and routines.

☐ Knowledge of my barriers and the tools to remove them.

☐ Support. (Mentor, Counselor, Parent, etc.)

☐ Personal Affirmations.

☐ Knowledge of my strengths and superpowers.

☐ My favorite pens, markers, highlighters, and stickers.

☐ A personal journal.

☐ The perfect planner.

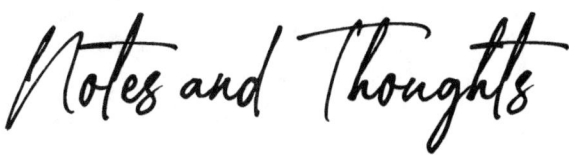

Notes

Notes

Notes

_____

_____

_____

_____

_____

_____

_____

_____

_____

_____

_____

_____

_____

_____

_____

Notes

Notes

Notes

Notes

C. ZAKI ROSHELL

CONCLUSION
AND INVITATION

*Y*ou did it! You have completed the first step in becoming the CEO of your self-confidence. With these tools you can move forward and continue to practice the strategies you've learned in this book.

I invite you to check out the planner I've created. It is the perfect companion to this book and was created with you in mind.

Visit www.zakiblaque.store

- Purchase your Little Blaque Planner
- Share how you feel about Becoming a CEO of Self-Confidence
- Read what others are saying
- Communicate with the Author

- • Purchase additional copies of Becoming a CEO of Self-Confidence for friends

For information about having the author speak to your organization or group, please contact: Pamela Roshell **prmanager@zakiblaque.store**

ACKNOWLEDGMENTS

The saying "it takes a village" has truly been experienced through this book project. My village includes my parents, Win and Pamela Roshell along with my GaMa, Angie Porter, who together are my forever cheerleaders and solid foundation. You never get in the way of me becoming me, thank you for encouraging me to grow as a young lady and as an entrepreneur.

I am grateful for my village of extended family and friends whose encouragement continues to be a source of inspiration. I want to express special thanks and gratitude to Dr. Vernard Hodges for providing the words in my foreword. In spite of your brutal schedule, you made time for me. My village of accountability and technical support, Terri King Hunt, the best writing coach, and the oh-so-amazing marketing guru, Tamara Zantell of Legacy Brand Creators.

Most of all, I want to thank God for vision, passion, and favor. I feel Your love daily.

REFERENCES

Bandura, A. (1977). Self-Efficacy: Toward a unifying Theory of Behavioral Change. Psychological Review, 84 (2), 191-215

Bergkvist, L. (2009). The Role of Confidence in Attitudes-Intention and Beliefs-Attitude Relationships. International Journal of Advertising, 28(5), 863-880

Goldberg, Lewis R. (1992). The Development of Markers for the Big-Five Factor Structure. Psychological assessment 4.1

Holland, J. L. (1958). A personality inventory employing occupational titles. Journal of Applied Psychology, 42, 336 - 342.

Miscisin, M. (2010). Showing our true colors (3rd edition). True Colors International.

Myers, I. (1962). The Myers Briggs type indicator: Manual. Palo Alto, CA: Consulting Psychologists Press.

Smalley, G. and Trent, J. (1999). The Two Sides of Love. Tyndale House Publishers, Carol Stream, Illinois

Personality Test for Teens:

> *https:llpersonalityacademy.com/wp-contentluploadsl2021l081Personality-Assessment-for-Teens.pdf*

Five Minute Personality Test:

> https://www.decal.ga.gov/documents/attachments/5minutepersonalitytest.pdf

The Big Five Personality Test:

> https://openpsychometrics.org/printable/big-five-personality-test.pdf

The Holland Code Test:

> https://openpsychometrics.org/printable/holland-code-test.pdf

The True Color Personality:

> https://sfp.caltech.edu/documents/4296/the mentoring spectrum true color test.pdf

ABOUT THE AUTHOR

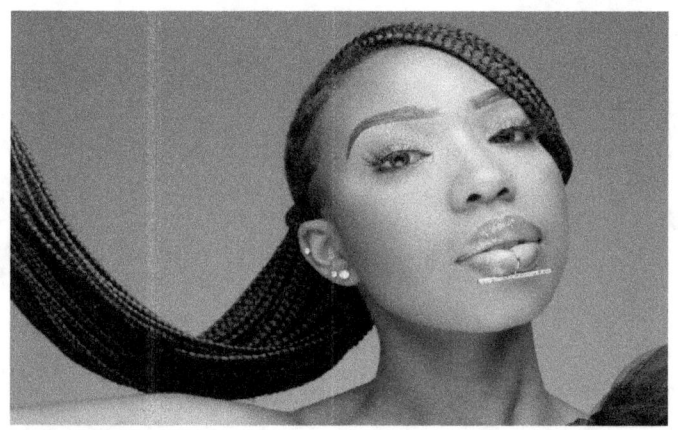

Zaki Roshell is a teen fashion designer and boutique owner from the great state of Georgia. As the CEO and founder of Zaki's Tutu Tops, she is on a mission to encourage young women to embrace their unique style and dare to make a statement.

Trained and certified in the art of public speaking, Zaki is leading a movement to encourage young people to live life with confidence and on their own terms. She is on a mission to remind young people that they are the CEOs of their life and that they should live that life with strength and passion.

In her spare time, Zaki enjoys traveling, snuggling with her pet Yorkie, Coco Cake, and creating new style designs through upcycling and vintage shopping.

www.ingramcontent.com/pod-product-compliance
Lightning Source LLC
Chambersburg PA
CBHW070719130626
46553CB00005B/2061